Wholesome

DELIGHTS

AT HOME

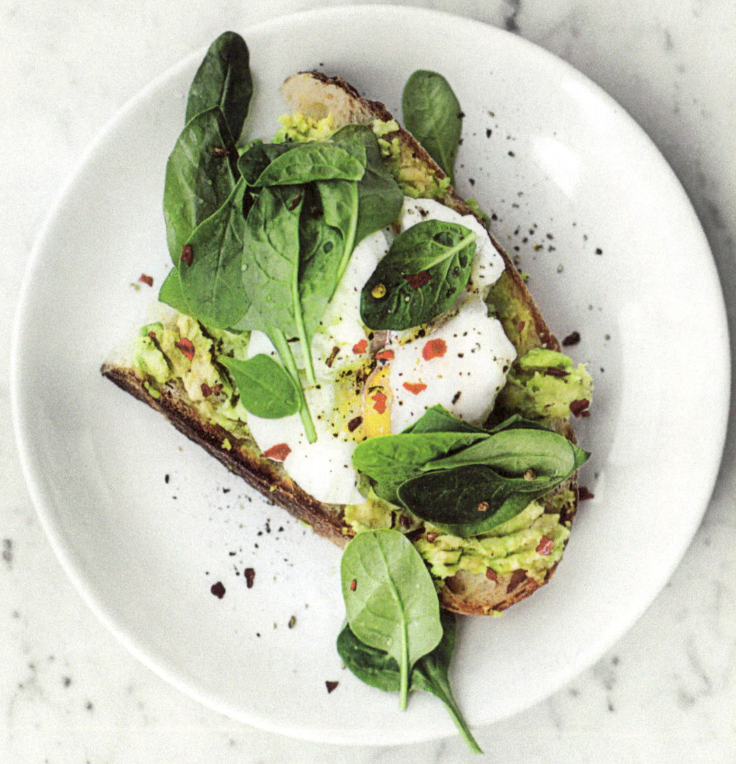

VOL. 1

CONTENTS

About me

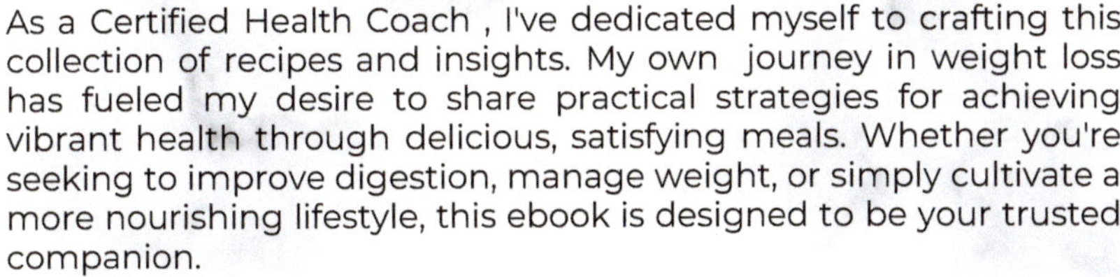

Welcome to Wholesome Delights,
where health and flavor converge to
redefine how you nourish your body and
delight your palate.
 I'm Angel Rae Vigil, passionate about
empowering individuals like you to embrace a wholesome approach
to eating that supports both wellness and enjoyment.

As a Certified Health Coach , I've dedicated myself to crafting this
collection of recipes and insights. My own journey in weight loss
has fueled my desire to share practical strategies for achieving
vibrant health through delicious, satisfying meals. Whether you're
seeking to improve digestion, manage weight, or simply cultivate a
more nourishing lifestyle, this ebook is designed to be your trusted
companion.

In "Wholesome Delights," you'll discover a treasure trove of recipes
that celebrate fresh, nutrient-dense ingredients and innovative
flavors. Each recipe is crafted with care, ensuring that every bite not
only supports your health goals but also brings joy to your kitchen.
Join me on this journey to transform the way you eat, one
wholesome recipe at a time. Let's embark together on a path
where food is not just fuel, but a source of vitality and pleasure.
Together, we'll create a healthier, happier you.
Thank you for choosing "Wholesome Delights" to guide you toward
a life filled with delicious and nutritious possibilities.

Xoxo,

Angel Rae Vigil

INTRO

Welcome to "Wholesome Delights," where nourishing your body and tantalizing your taste buds go hand in hand! This ebook is your guide to a journey of culinary exploration, packed with mouthwatering recipes that are not only delicious but also support your goals of losing weight and enhancing gut health. Get ready to embark on a flavorful adventure that will leave you feeling energized, satisfied, and rejuvenated!

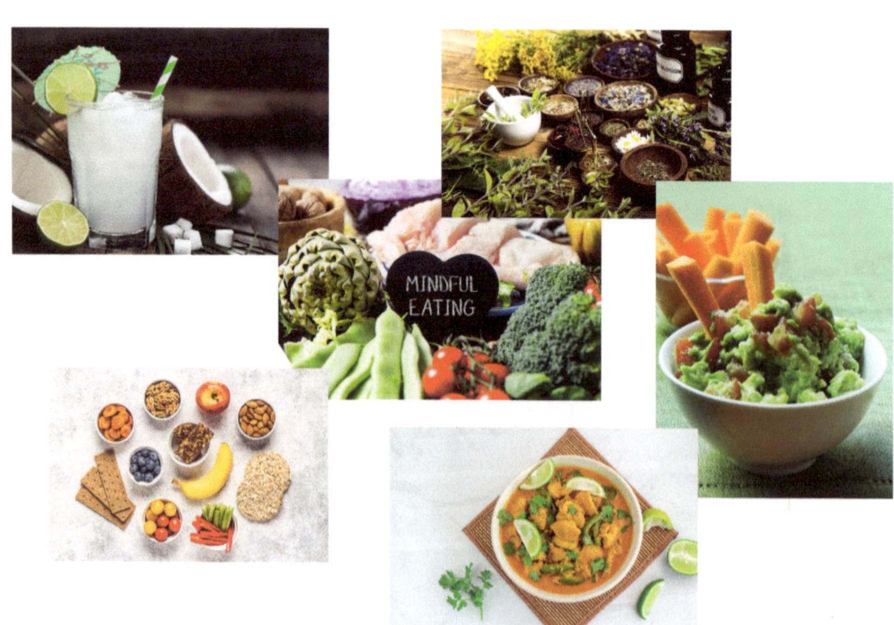

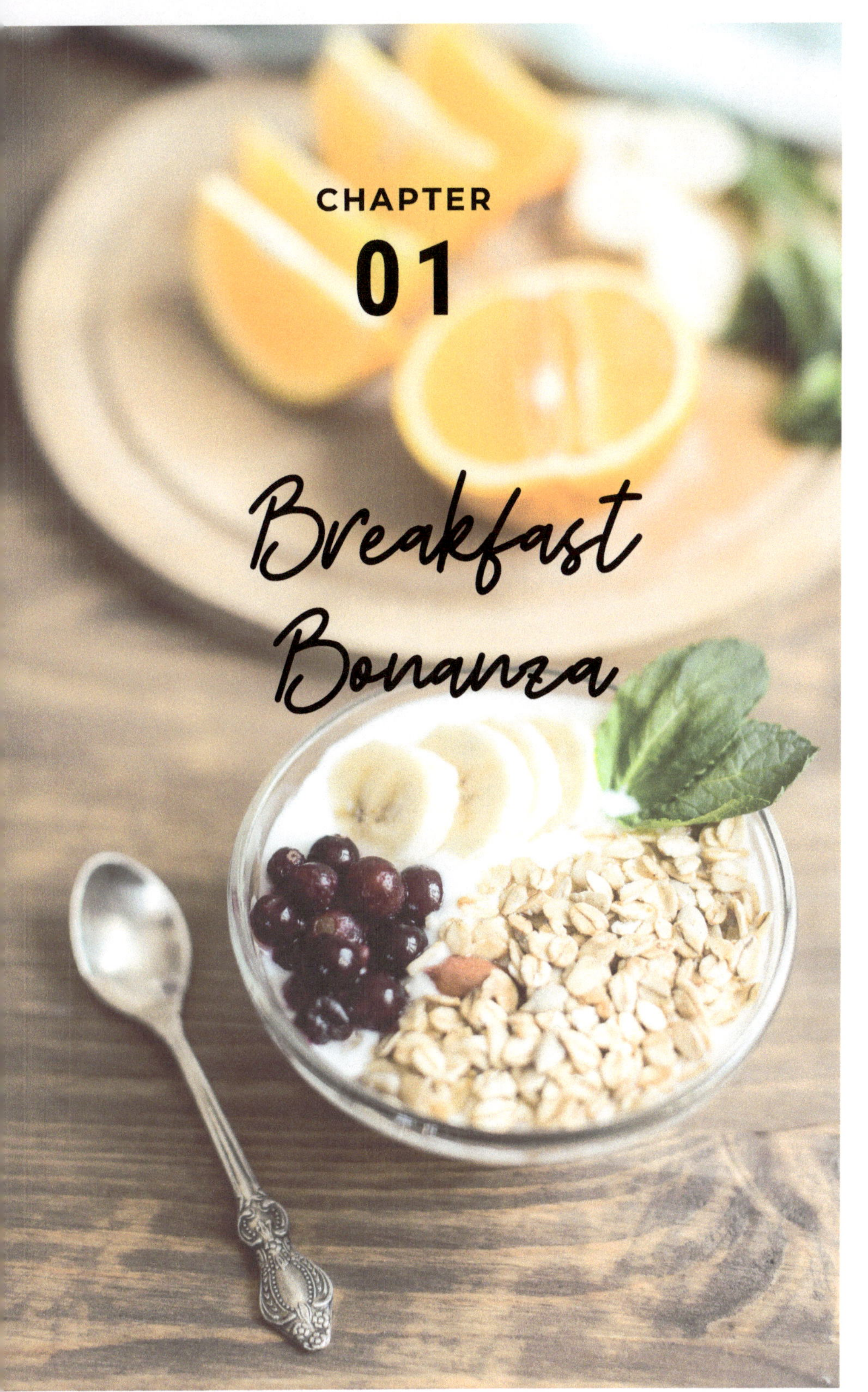
CHAPTER
01
Breakfast
Bonanza

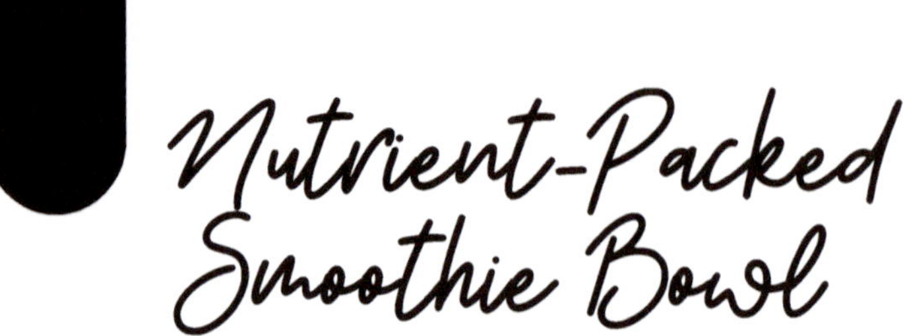

Nutrient-Packed Smoothie Bowl

INGREDIENTS

- 1 frozen banana
- 1 cup mixed berries (such as strawberries, blueberries, and raspberries)
- 1/2 cup spinach or kale
- 1/2 cup almond milk (or any dairy-free milk of choice)
- 1 tablespoon chia seeds
- Toppings: sliced fresh fruits, nuts, seeds, granola, coconut flakes

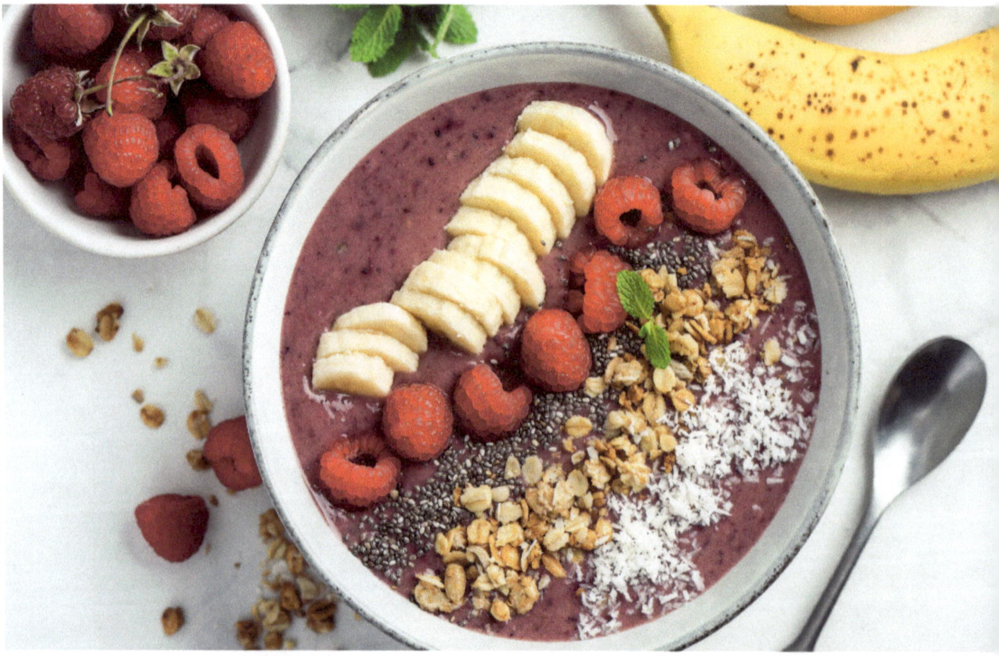

01 Nutrient-Packed Smoothie Bowl

INSTRUCTIONS

1. In a blender, combine the frozen banana, mixed berries, spinach or kale, almond milk, and chia seeds.
2. Blend until smooth and creamy, adding more almond milk if needed to reach your desired consistency.
3. Pour the smoothie into a bowl and top with your favorite toppings, such as sliced fresh fruits, nuts, seeds, granola, and coconut flakes.
4. Enjoy your nutrient-packed smoothie bowl for a refreshing and energizing start to your day!

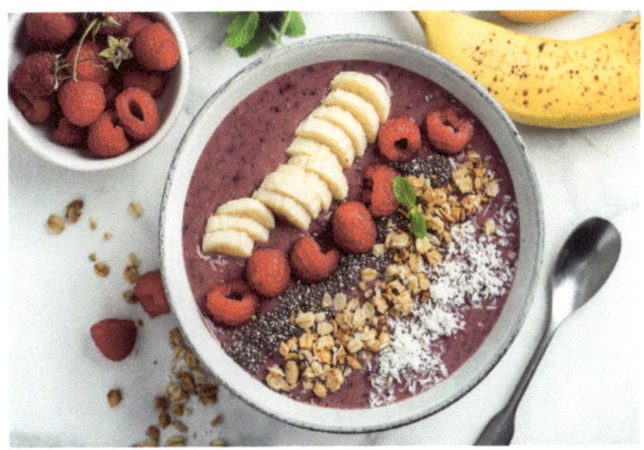

01 Tropical paradise Smoothie

INGREDIENTS

- 1/2 cup frozen pineapple chunks
- 1/2 cup frozen mango chunks
- 1/2 cup coconut milk (or any dairy-free milk of choice)
- 1/4 cup Greek yogurt (or dairy-free yogurt for a vegan option)
- 1 tablespoon honey or maple syrup (optional, for sweetness)
- Juice of 1/2 lime
- Toppings: shredded coconut, sliced kiwi, diced mango, chia seeds

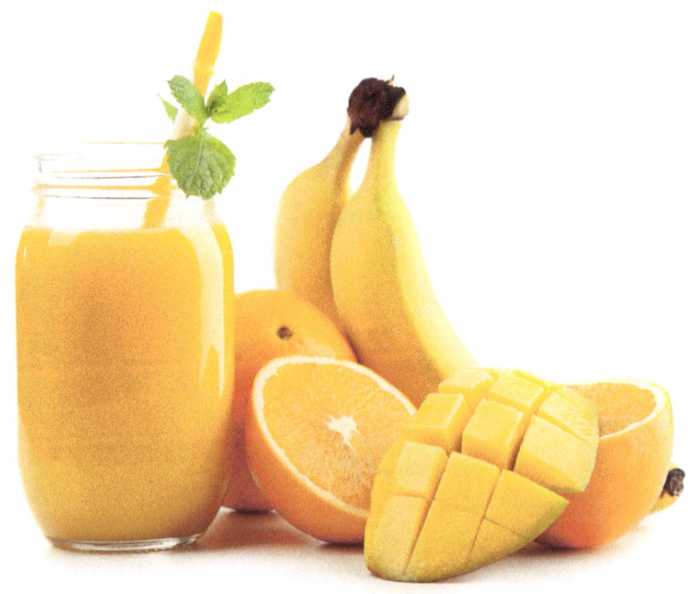

01 Tropical paradise Smoothie

INSTRUCTIONS

1. In a blender, combine the frozen pineapple chunks, frozen mango chunks, coconut milk, Greek yogurt, honey or maple syrup (if using), and lime juice.
2. Blend until smooth and creamy.
3. Pour the smoothie into a glass and garnish with shredded coconut, sliced kiwi, diced mango, and chia seeds.
4. Serve immediately and transport yourself to a tropical paradise with every sip!

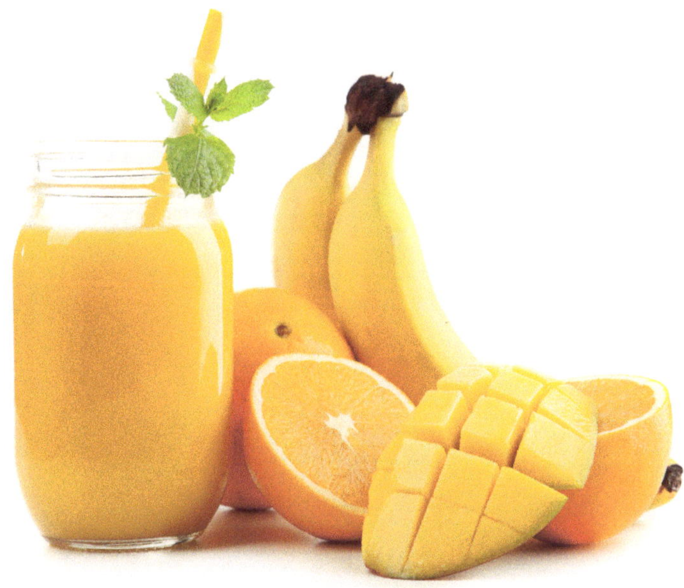

01 *Sweet Potato Hash*

INGREDIENTS

- 1 large sweet potato, peeled and diced into small cubes
- 1 bell pepper, diced
- 1 small red onion, diced
- 2 cloves garlic, minced
- 2 tablespoons olive oil
- 1 teaspoon smoked paprika
- 1/2 teaspoon ground cumin
- Salt and pepper to taste
- 4 eggs
- Fresh cilantro, chopped (for garnish, optional)
- Avocado slices (for serving, optional)

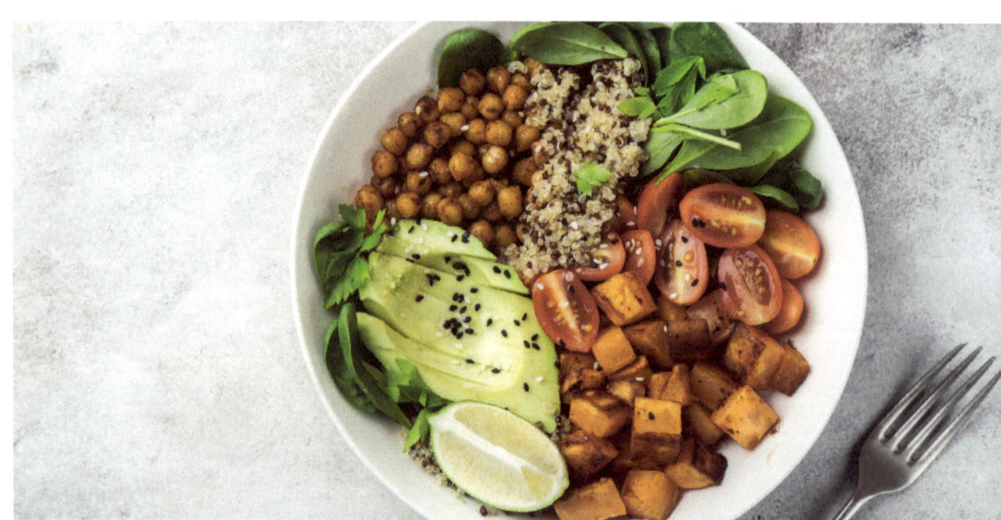

01 Sweet Potato Hash

INSTRUCTIONS

1. Heat the olive oil in a large skillet over medium heat. Add the diced sweet potato and cook for 5-7 minutes, stirring occasionally, until slightly softened.
2. Add the diced bell pepper, red onion, and minced garlic to the skillet. Cook for another 5-7 minutes, or until the vegetables are tender.
3. Sprinkle the smoked paprika, ground cumin, salt, and pepper over the vegetables. Stir to combine and cook for an additional 1-2 minutes to allow the spices to toast.
4. Create four small wells in the hash mixture and crack an egg into each well. Cover the skillet and cook for 5-7 minutes, or until the egg whites are set but the yolks are still runny.
5. Once the eggs are cooked to your liking, remove the skillet from the heat. Garnish with fresh cilantro, if desired, and serve with avocado slices on the side.

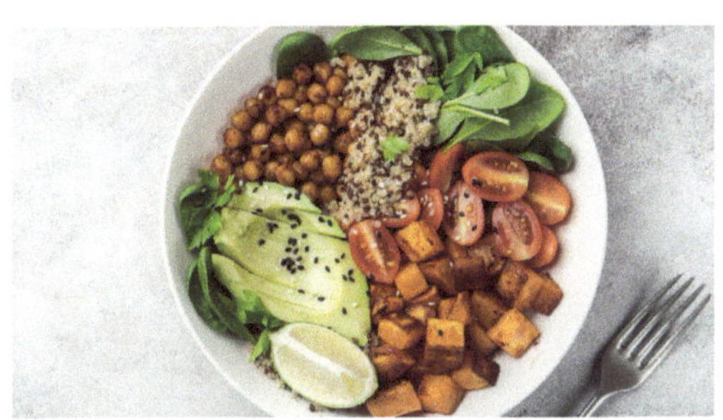

01 Coconut Chia pudding

INGREDIENTS

- 1/4 cup chia seeds
- 1 cup coconut milk (or any dairy-free milk of choice)
- 1 tablespoon maple syrup or honey (optional, for sweetness)
- 1/2 teaspoon vanilla extract
- Mixed berries (such as strawberries, blueberries, raspberries)
- Toasted coconut flakes (for garnish, optional)
- Fresh mint leaves (for garnish, optional)

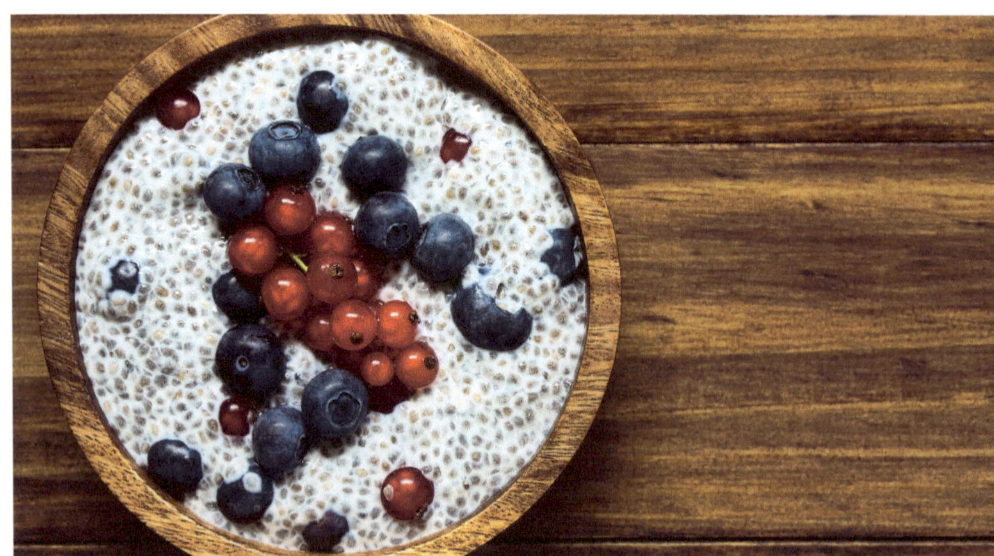

01 Coconut Chia pudding

INSTRUCTIONS

- In a bowl or jar, combine the chia seeds, coconut milk, maple syrup or honey (if using), and vanilla extract. Stir well to combine.
- Cover the bowl or jar and refrigerate for at least 4 hours or overnight, allowing the chia seeds to absorb the liquid and thicken into a pudding-like consistency.
- Once the chia pudding has set, give it a good stir. If it's too thick, you can add a splash of coconut milk to reach your desired consistency.
- Spoon the chia pudding into serving bowls or glasses. Top with mixed berries and sprinkle with toasted coconut flakes, if desired.
- Garnish with fresh mint leaves for a pop of color and freshness.
- Serve chilled and enjoy this creamy, coconutty delight for a sweet and satisfying breakfast!

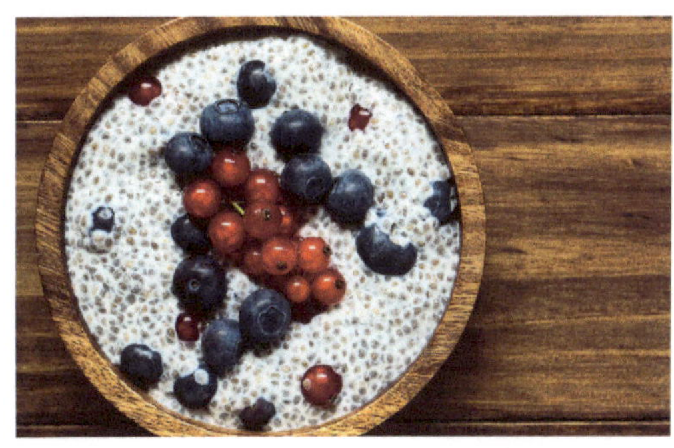

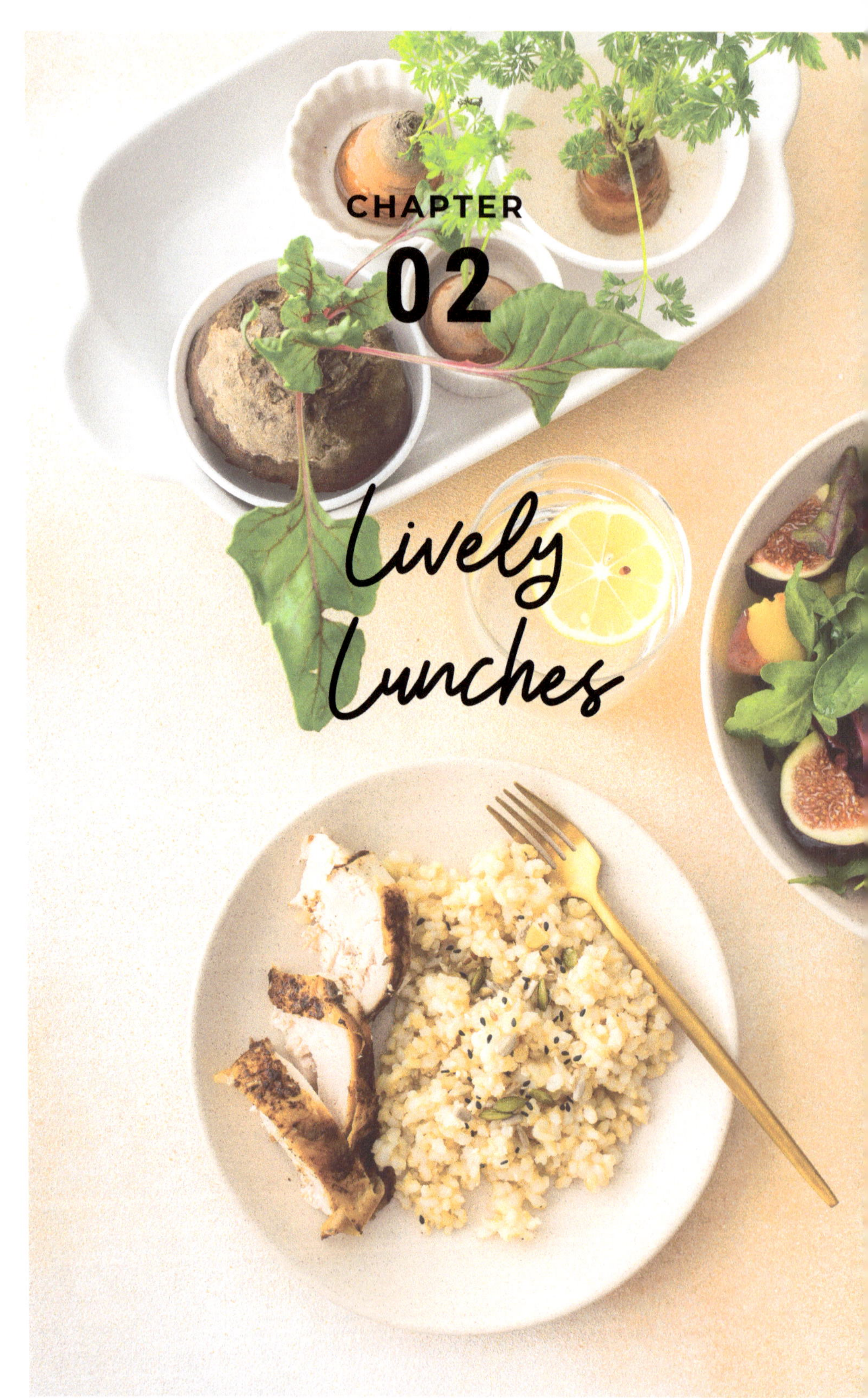
CHAPTER
02
Lively
Lunches

LIVELY LUNCHES

Wave goodbye to dull lunches and embrace these vibrant, nourishing meal ideas. Whether you're in the mood for a revitalizing salad, a comforting bowl of soup, or a fulfilling wrap, you'll discover an array of choices to excite your palate and keep you energized until dinnertime.

02 Grilled Chicken & Quinoa Salad

INGREDIENTS

- 1 cup quinoa, rinsed
- 2 cups water or chicken broth
- 2 chicken breasts, grilled and diced
- 1 red bell pepper, diced
- 1 cucumber, diced
- 1/4 red onion, thinly sliced
- 1/4 cup fresh parsley, chopped
- Juice of 1 lemon
- 2 tablespoons olive oil
- Salt and pepper to taste

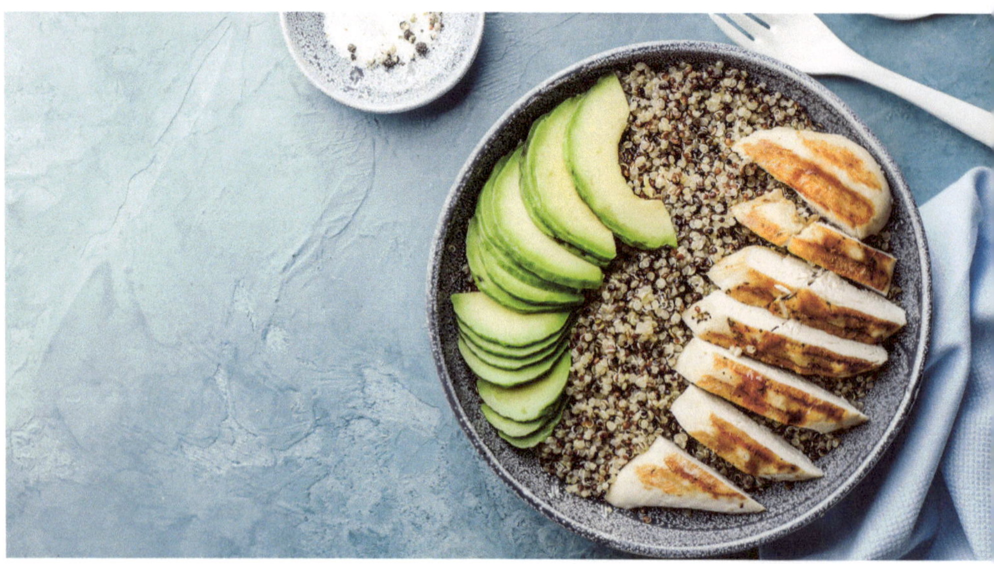

02 Grilled Chicken & Quinoa Salad

INSTRUCTIONS

1. In a medium saucepan, bring the water or broth to a boil. Add quinoa, reduce heat to low, cover, and simmer for 15 minutes or until quinoa is cooked and liquid is absorbed. Remove from heat and let it cool.
2. In a large bowl, combine cooked quinoa, grilled chicken, red bell pepper, cucumber, red onion, and parsley.
3. In a small bowl, whisk together lemon juice, olive oil, salt, and pepper. Pour over the salad and toss gently to combine.
4. Serve immediately or divide into meal prep containers for lunches throughout the week.

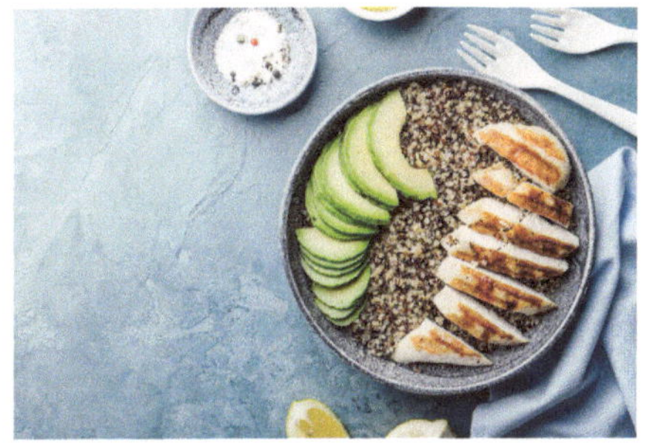

02 Sweet Potato & Chickpea Buddha Bowl

INGREDIENTS

- 2 medium sweet potatoes, peeled and cubed
- 1 can (15 oz) chickpeas, rinsed and drained
- 1 tablespoon olive oil
- 1 teaspoon paprika
- 1/2 teaspoon cumin
- Salt and pepper to taste
- 2 cups cooked quinoa or brown rice
- 2 cups baby spinach or mixed greens
- 1 avocado, sliced
- Tahini dressing (store-bought or homemade)

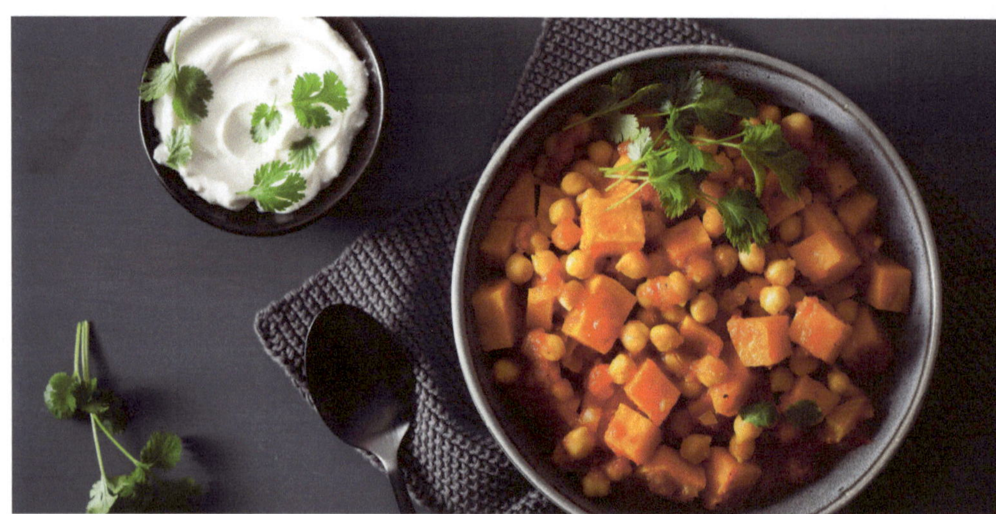

Sweet Potato & Chickpea Buddha Bowl

INSTRUCTIONS

1. Preheat oven to 400°F (200°C). Line a baking sheet with parchment paper.
2. In a bowl, toss sweet potatoes and chickpeas with olive oil, paprika, cumin, salt, and pepper. Spread evenly on the baking sheet.
3. Roast for 25-30 minutes, stirring halfway through, until sweet potatoes are tender and chickpeas are crispy.
4. Divide quinoa or brown rice among bowls. Top with roasted sweet potatoes and chickpeas, baby spinach or mixed greens, avocado slices, and drizzle with tahini dressing.
5. Enjoy immediately, or pack into meal prep containers for a satisfying lunch.

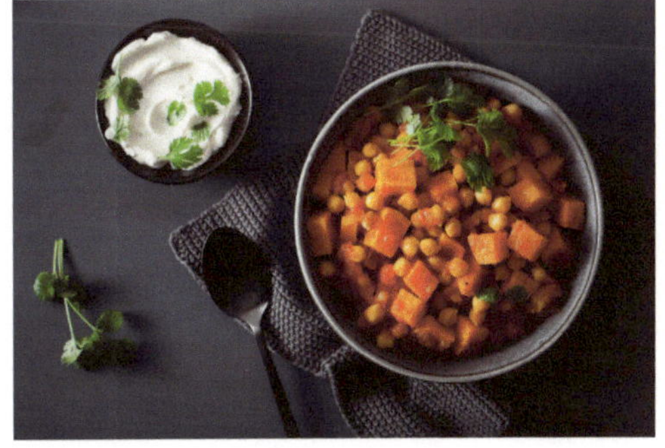

02 Chicken & Vegetable Stir-Fry

INGREDIENTS

- 2 chicken breasts, thinly sliced
- 2 tablespoons coconut aminos (or gluten-free soy sauce)
- 1 tablespoon sesame oil
- 1 tablespoon olive oil
- 2 garlic cloves, minced
- 1 inch fresh ginger, minced
- 1 red bell pepper, sliced
- 1 cup broccoli florets
- 1 carrot, julienned
- 1/2 cup snap peas
- Salt and pepper to taste

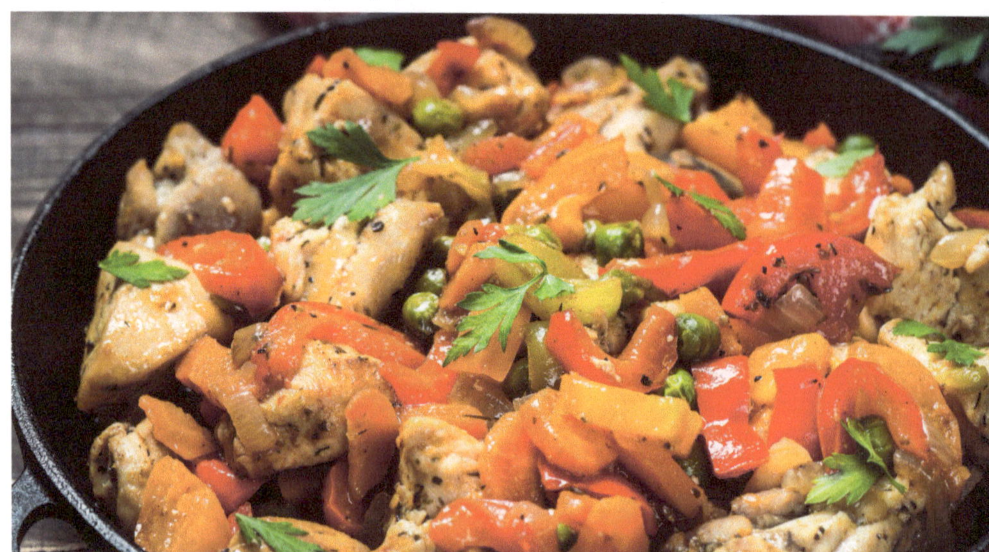

Chicken & Vegetable Stir-Fry

INSTRUCTIONS

1. In a bowl, marinate chicken slices with coconut aminos (or soy sauce) for 10 minutes.
2. Heat olive oil and sesame oil in a large skillet or wok over medium-high heat. Add garlic and ginger, sauté for 1 minute until fragrant.
3. Add marinated chicken slices to the skillet. Stir-fry for 5-6 minutes until chicken is cooked through.
4. Add bell pepper, broccoli, carrot, and snap peas to the skillet. Stir-fry for another 3-4 minutes until vegetables are tender-crisp.
5. Season with salt and pepper to taste. Serve immediately over cooked rice or cauliflower rice, or divide into meal prep containers for later.

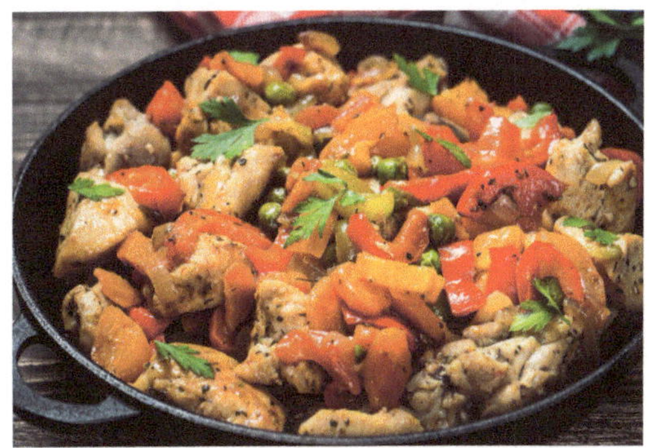

Chicken & Avocado Wrap

INGREDIENTS

- 2 large gluten-free wraps
- 1 avocado, mashed
- 1 cup cooked chicken, shredded
- 1/2 cup cherry tomatoes, halved
- 1/4 cup cucumber, thinly sliced
- Handful of baby spinach or mixed greens
- Hummus or dairy-free spread of choice of rice

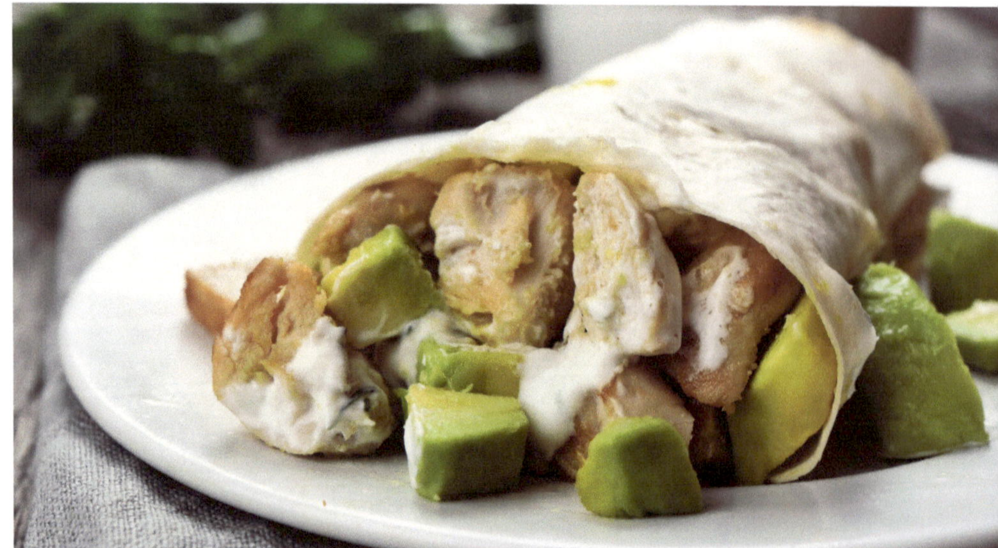

02 Chicken & Avocado Wrap

INSTRUCTIONS

1. Lay out gluten-free wraps on a clean surface. Spread mashed avocado evenly over each wrap.
2. Layer shredded chicken, cherry tomatoes, cucumber slices, and baby spinach or mixed greens on top of the avocado spread.
3. Drizzle with hummus or dairy-free spread of choice.
4. Roll up wraps tightly, folding in the sides as you go.
5. Slice in half and enjoy immediately, or wrap tightly in plastic wrap and refrigerate for a quick grab-and-go lunch.

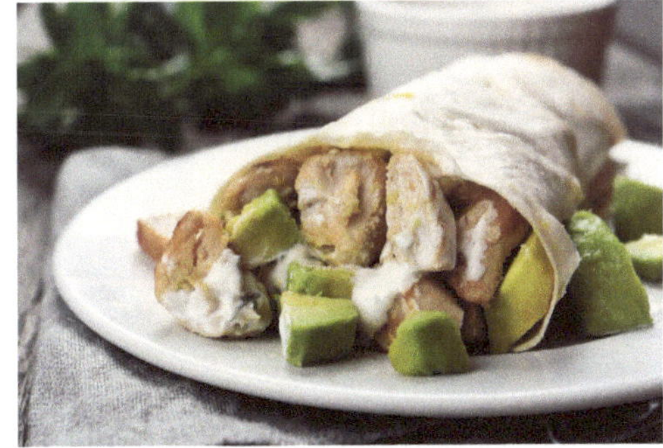

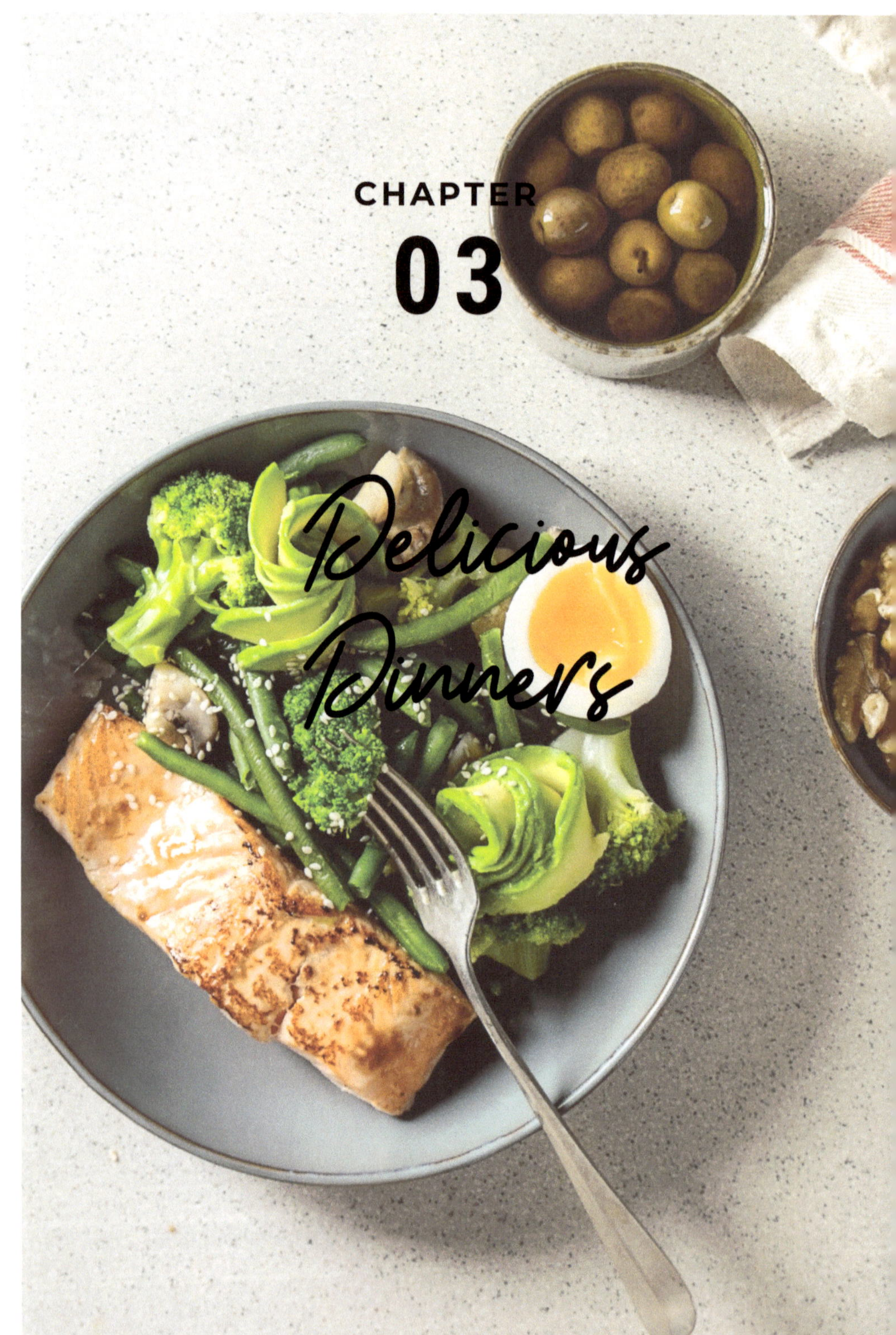

Delicious Dinners

03 Baked Lemon Garlic Chicken with Roasted Vegetables

INGREDIENTS

- 4 boneless, skinless chicken breasts
- 2 tablespoons olive oil
- Juice and zest of 1 lemon
- 3 cloves garlic, minced
- 1 teaspoon dried oregano
- 1 teaspoon dried thyme
- Salt and pepper to taste
- 1 pound baby potatoes, halved
- 1 bunch asparagus, trimmed
- 1 red bell pepper, sliced
- Fresh parsley for garnish

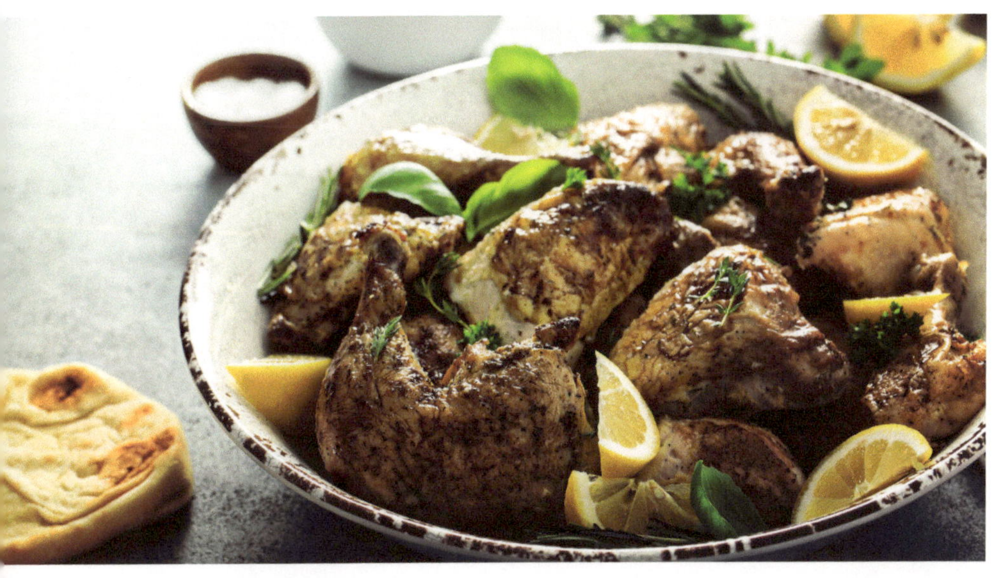

03 Baked Lemon Garlic Chicken with Roasted Vegetables

INSTRUCTIONS

1. Preheat oven to 400°F (200°C). Line a baking sheet with parchment paper.
2. In a small bowl, whisk together olive oil, lemon juice and zest, minced garlic, oregano, thyme, salt, and pepper.
3. Place chicken breasts on the prepared baking sheet. Brush both sides with the lemon garlic mixture.
4. In a separate bowl, toss baby potatoes, asparagus, and red bell pepper with remaining lemon garlic mixture. Arrange vegetables around the chicken on the baking sheet.
5. Bake for 20-25 minutes, or until chicken is cooked through (internal temperature of 165°F or 74°C) and vegetables are tender.
6. Garnish with fresh parsley and serve hot

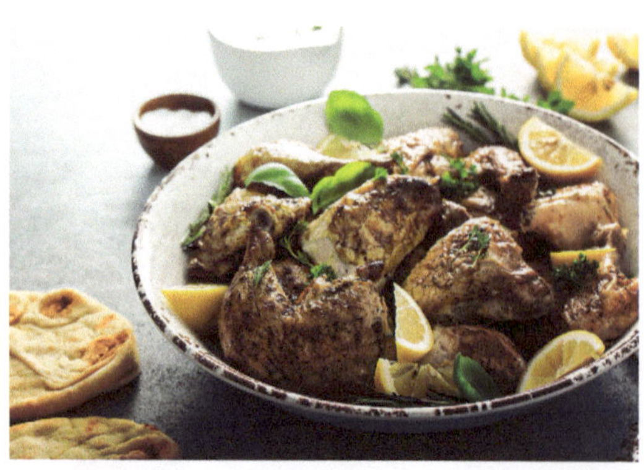

Quinoa Stuffed Bell Peppers

03

INGREDIENTS

- 4 large bell peppers, tops cut off and seeds removed
- 1 cup quinoa, rinsed
- 2 cups vegetable broth or water
- 1 tablespoon olive oil
- 1 onion, diced
- 2 cloves garlic, minced
- 1 zucchini, diced
- 1 cup diced tomatoes (canned or fresh)
- 1 teaspoon dried oregano
- 1 teaspoon paprika
- Salt and pepper to taste
- Fresh basil for garnish

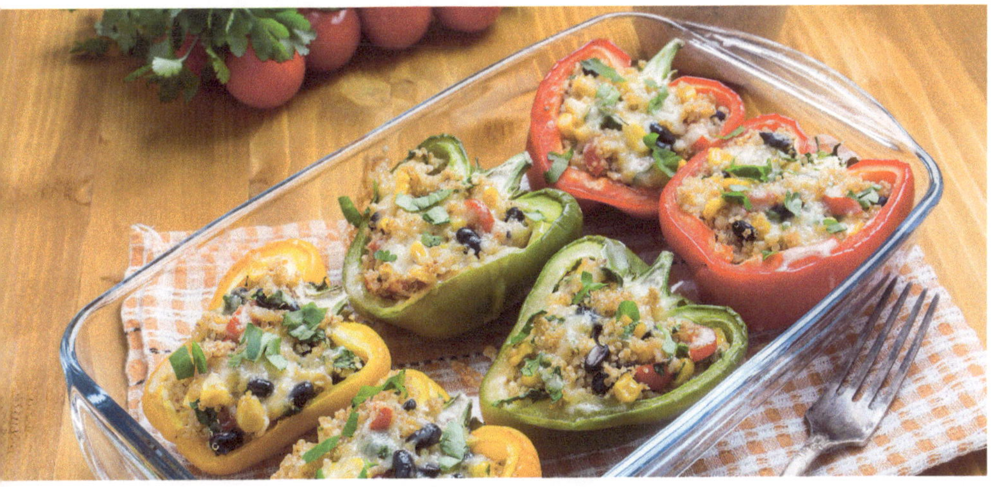

03 Quinoa Stuffed Bell Peppers

INSTRUCTIONS

1. Preheat oven to 375°F (190°C). Place the hollowed-out bell peppers in a baking dish.
2. In a medium saucepan, bring vegetable broth (or water) to a boil. Add quinoa, reduce heat to low, cover, and simmer for 15 minutes or until quinoa is cooked and liquid is absorbed.
3. In a large skillet, heat olive oil over medium heat. Add onion and garlic, sauté until softened and fragrant.
4. Add diced zucchini, tomatoes, oregano, paprika, salt, and pepper to the skillet. Cook for 5-7 minutes until vegetables are tender.
5. Stir cooked quinoa into the vegetable mixture. Adjust seasoning if needed.
6. Spoon quinoa mixture evenly into the bell peppers.
7. Cover the baking dish with foil and bake for 25-30 minutes, or until peppers are tender.
8. Garnish with fresh basil before serving.

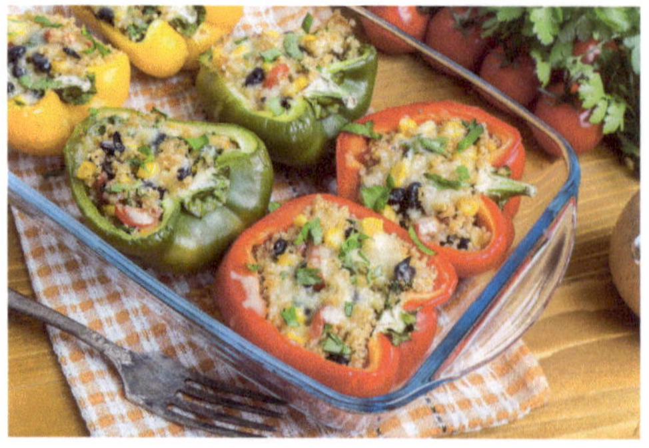

03 Thai Coconut Curry with Chicken and Vegetables

INGREDIENTS

- 2 tablespoons coconut oil
- 1 onion, thinly sliced
- 3 cloves garlic, minced
- 1 red bell pepper, sliced
- 1 carrot, thinly sliced
- 1 zucchini, sliced
- 1 pound boneless, skinless chicken thighs, cut into bite-sized pieces
- 2 tablespoons Thai red curry paste
- 1 can (14 oz) coconut milk
- 1 tablespoon fish sauce (optional, for added depth of flavor)
- Juice of 1 lime
- Salt and pepper to taste
- Fresh cilantro for garnish
- Cooked rice or rice noodles

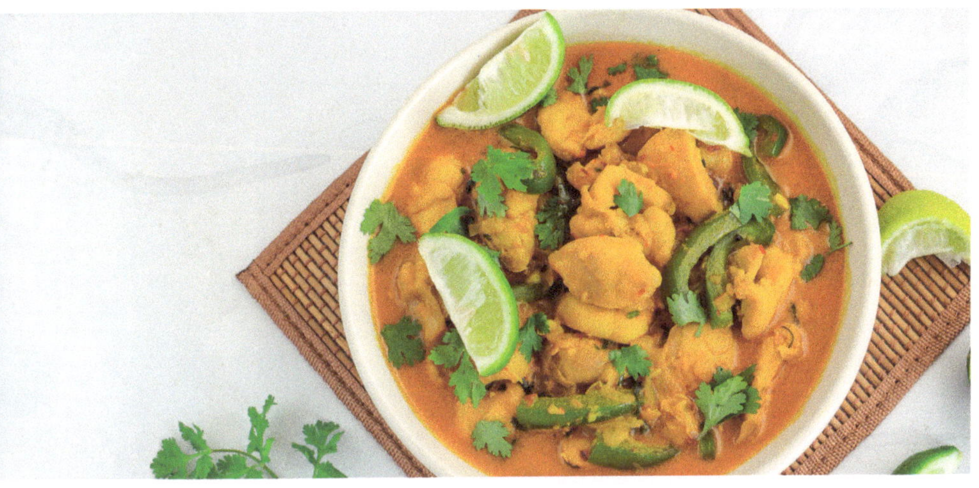

Thai Coconut Curry with Chicken and Vegetables

03

INSTRUCTIONS

1. In a large skillet or wok, heat coconut oil over medium-high heat. Add sliced onion and garlic, sauté until softened and fragrant.
2. Add red bell pepper, carrot, and zucchini to the skillet. Stir-fry for 3-4 minutes until vegetables start to soften.
3. Push vegetables to the side of the skillet and add chicken pieces to the center. Cook until chicken is browned on all sides.
4. Stir in Thai red curry paste and cook for 1 minute until fragrant.
5. Pour in coconut milk and fish sauce (if using). Bring to a simmer and cook for 10-12 minutes, stirring occasionally, until chicken is cooked through and vegetables are tender.
6. Stir in lime juice, season with salt and pepper to taste.
7. Serve hot over cooked rice or rice noodles. Garnish with fresh cilantro.

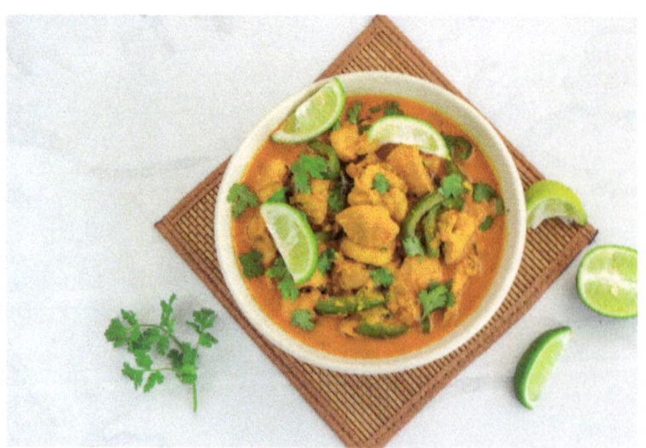

03 — Mediterranean Grilled Chicken Salad

INGREDIENTS

- 2 chicken breasts
- 2 tablespoons olive oil
- 1 teaspoon dried oregano
- 1 teaspoon dried basil
- Salt and pepper to taste
- 4 cups mixed greens (such as spinach, arugula, and romaine)
- 1 cucumber, sliced
- 1 cup cherry tomatoes, halved
- 1/4 red onion, thinly sliced
- 1/4 cup Kalamata olives, sliced
- 1/4 cup crumbled dairy-free feta cheese (optional)
- Lemon wedges for serving
- Balsamic vinaigrette (store-bought or homemade)

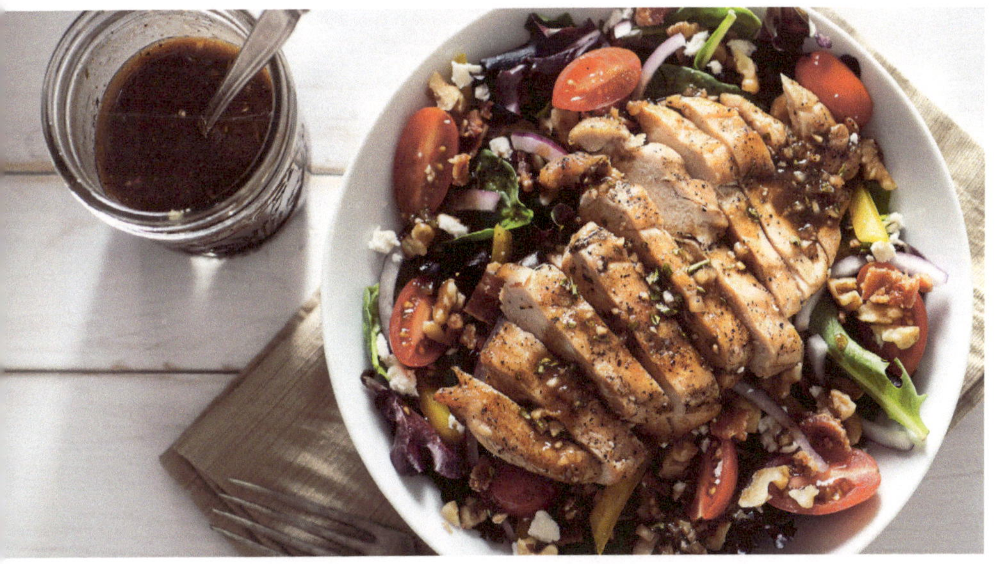

Mediterranean Grilled Chicken Salad

INSTRUCTIONS

1. Preheat grill or grill pan over medium-high heat.
2. In a bowl, combine olive oil, dried oregano, dried basil, salt, and pepper. Brush both sides of chicken breasts with the mixture.
3. Grill chicken breasts for 5-7 minutes per side, or until cooked through (internal temperature of 165°F or 74°C). Remove from grill and let rest for a few minutes before slicing.
4. In a large salad bowl, arrange mixed greens, sliced cucumber, cherry tomatoes, red onion, and Kalamata olives.
5. Top the salad with sliced grilled chicken.
6. Sprinkle dairy-free feta cheese (if using) over the salad.
7. Serve with lemon wedges and drizzle with balsamic vinaigrette.

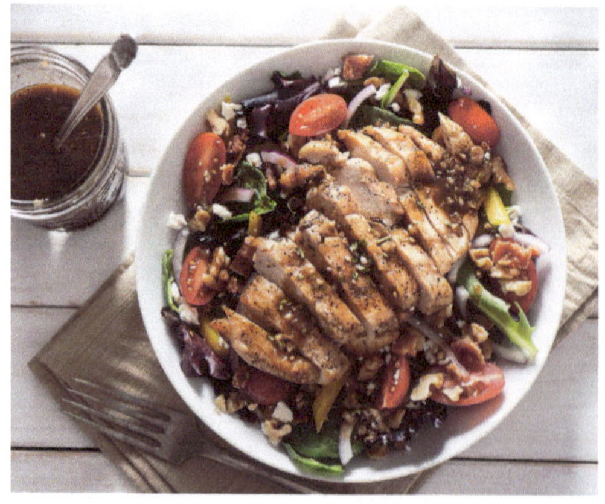

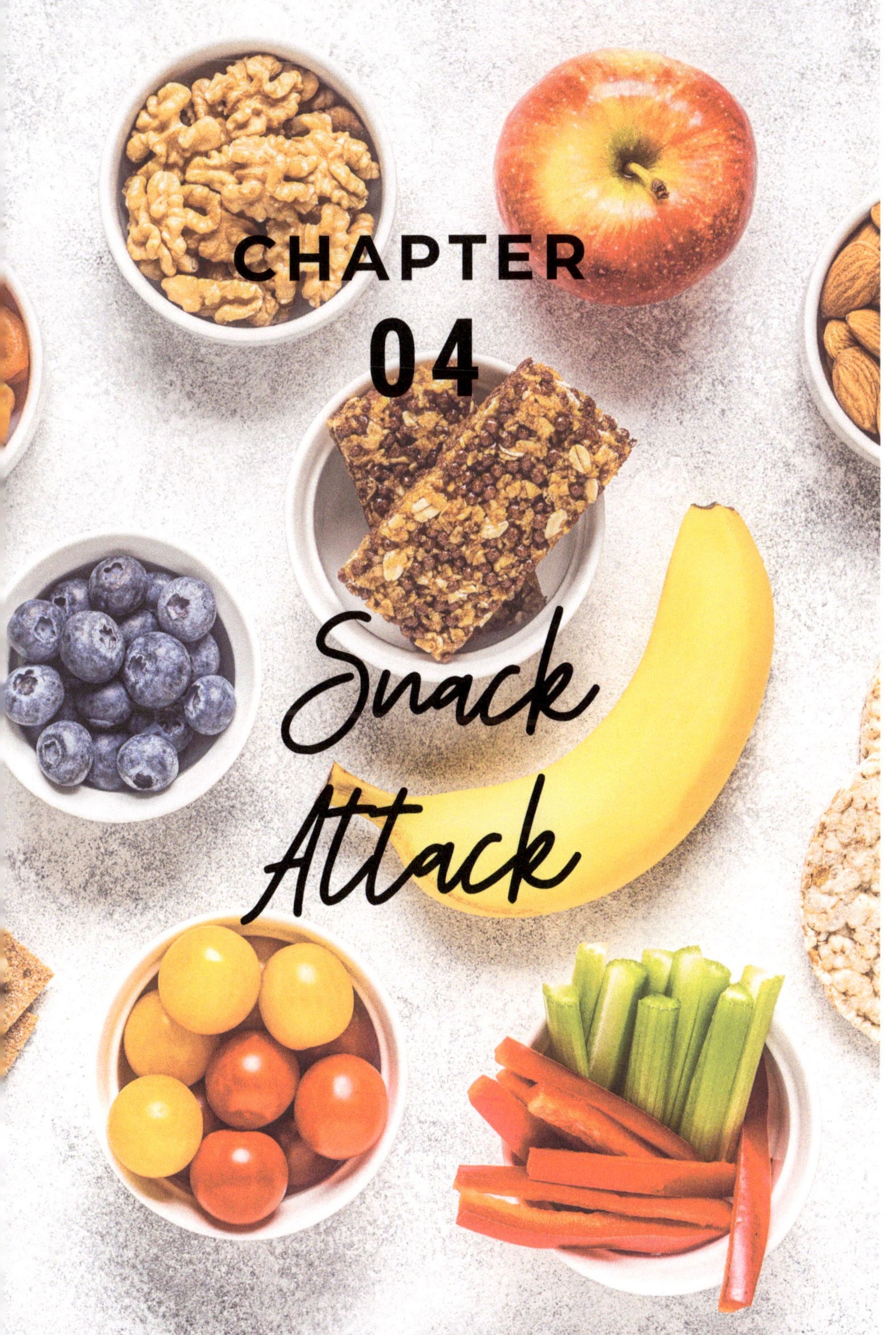
CHAPTER
04
Snack
Attack

04 — Mediterranean Hummus Platter

INGREDIENTS

- 1 cup homemade or store-bought hummus
- 1 cucumber, sliced
- 1 cup cherry tomatoes, halved
- 1/4 cup Kalamata olives
- Gluten-free crackers or carrot sticks for dipping

INSTRUCTIONS

- Arrange a serving platter or plate with a generous dollop of hummus in the center.
- Surround the hummus with cucumber slices, cherry tomatoes, and Kalamata olives.
- Serve with gluten-free crackers or carrot sticks for dipping.

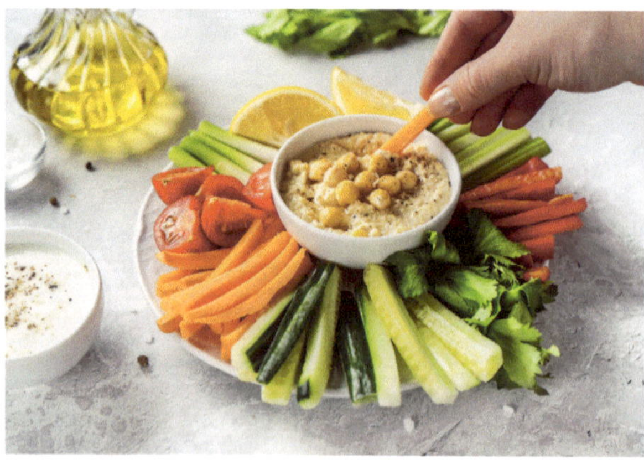

Apple Slices with Almond Butter

INGREDIENTS

- 2 apples, cored and sliced
- Almond butter (or any nut or seed butter of your choice)
- Optional toppings: chia seeds, hemp seeds, or sliced almonds

INSTRUCTIONS

- Arrange apple slices on a plate.
- Spread almond butter on each slice or serve it in a small bowl for dipping.
- Sprinkle with optional toppings like chia seeds, hemp seeds, or sliced almonds.

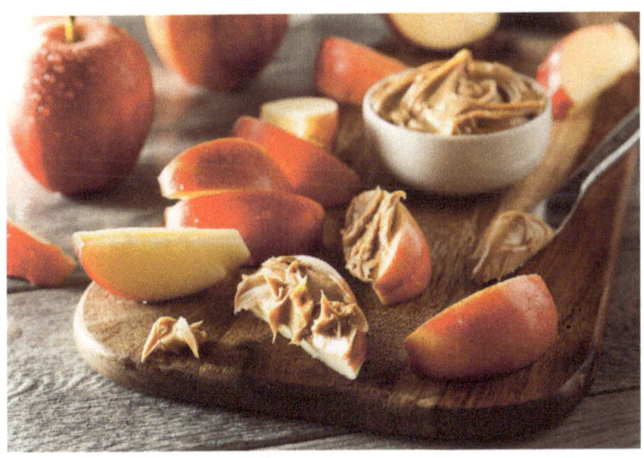

04 Trail Mix

INGREDIENTS

- 1 cup mixed nuts (almonds, cashews, walnuts, etc.)
- 1/2 cup dried fruit (raisins, cranberries, apricots, etc.)
- 1/4 cup dairy-free chocolate chips or cacao nibs (optional)

INSTRUCTIONS

- Combine mixed nuts, dried fruit, and dairy-free chocolate chips or cacao nibs in a bowl.
- Mix well to combine.
- Portion into small snack bags or containers for easy grab-and-go snacking.

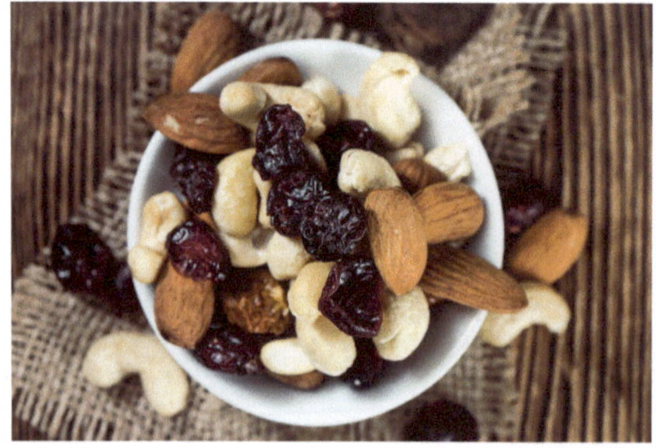

04 Veggie Sticks with Guacamole

INGREDIENTS

- 2 ripe avocados
- Juice of 1 lime
- 1/2 teaspoon garlic powder
- Salt and pepper to taste
- Assorted veggie sticks (carrots, celery, bell peppers, cucumber)

INSTRUCTIONS

- In a bowl, mash the ripe avocados with lime juice, garlic powder, salt, and pepper until smooth.
- Serve the guacamole with assorted veggie sticks for dipping.

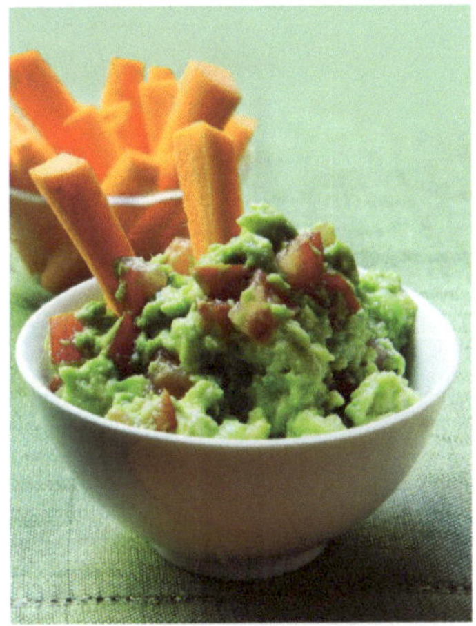

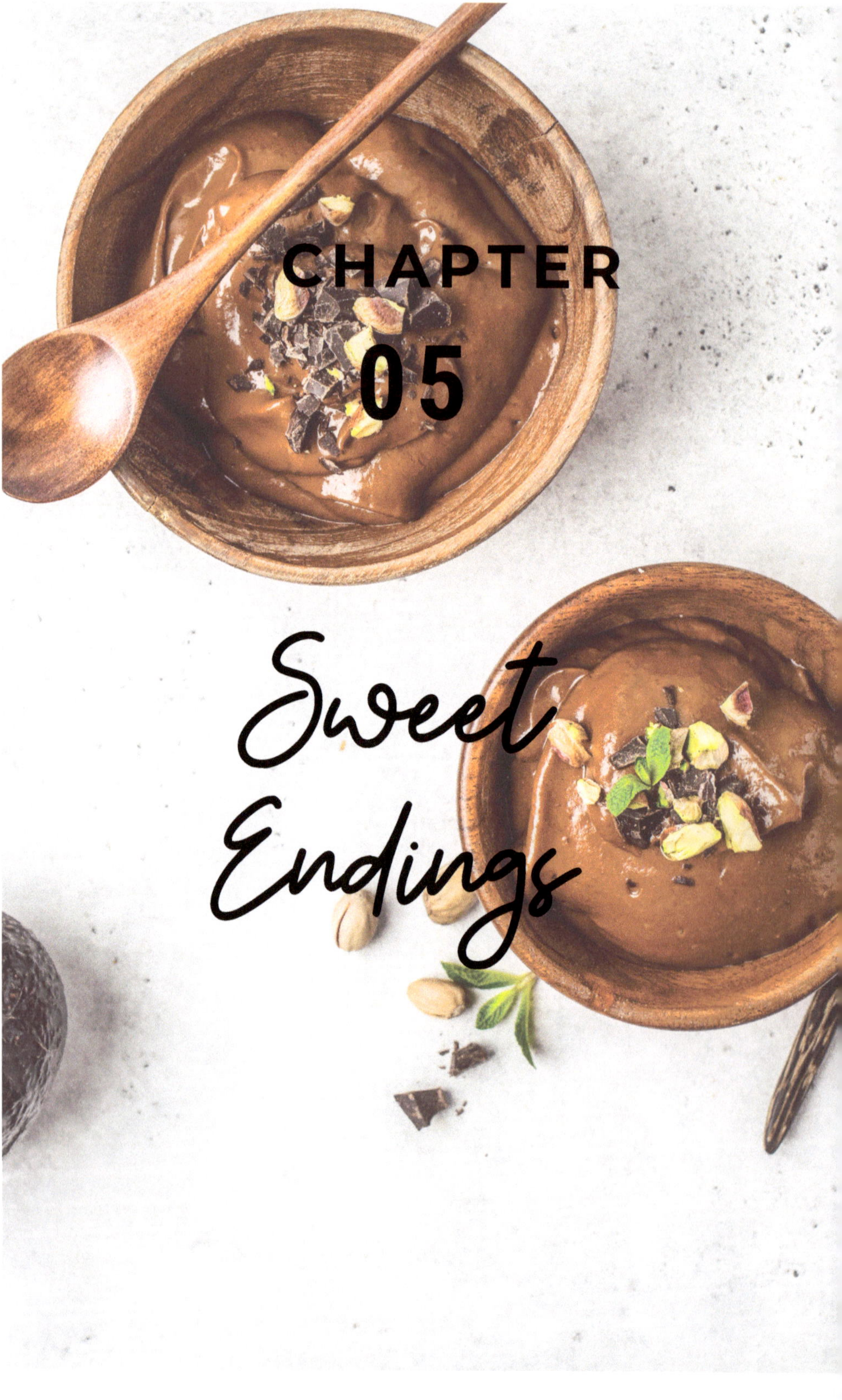

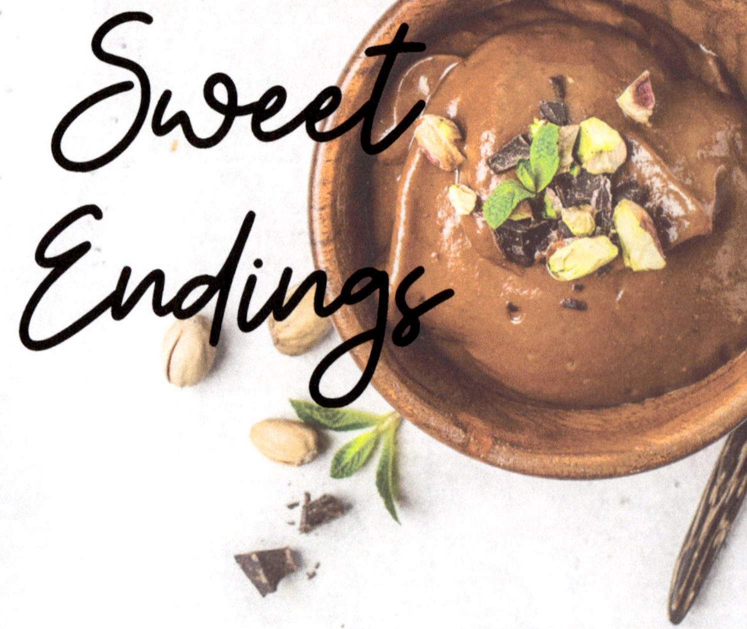

CHAPTER
05
Sweet
Endings

Coconut Mango Chia Pudding

INGREDIENTS

- 1/4 cup chia seeds
- 1 cup coconut milk (full-fat from a can)
- 1 tablespoon maple syrup (adjust to taste)
- 1/2 teaspoon vanilla extract
- 1 ripe mango, diced
- Unsweetened shredded coconut for garnish

INSTRUCTIONS

1. In a bowl, combine chia seeds, coconut milk, maple syrup, and vanilla extract. Stir well to combine.
2. Cover and refrigerate for at least 4 hours or overnight, until the mixture thickens into a pudding-like consistency.
3. In serving glasses or bowls, layer the chia pudding with diced mango.
4. Sprinkle with unsweetened shredded coconut before serving.

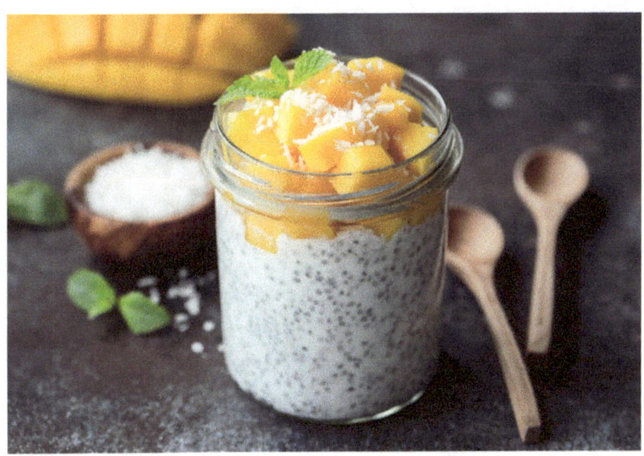

05 Chocolate Avocado Mousse

INGREDIENTS

- 2 ripe avocados
- 1/4 cup cocoa powder
- 1/4 cup maple syrup or agave syrup (adjust to taste)
- 1 teaspoon vanilla extract
- Pinch of salt
- Fresh berries for garnish

INSTRUCTIONS

1. Scoop the flesh of the avocados into a food processor or blender.
2. Add cocoa powder, maple syrup (or agave syrup), vanilla extract, and a pinch of salt.
3. Blend until smooth and creamy, scraping down the sides as needed.
4. Transfer to serving bowls or glasses.
5. Refrigerate for 30 minutes to chill.
6. Garnish with fresh berries before serving.

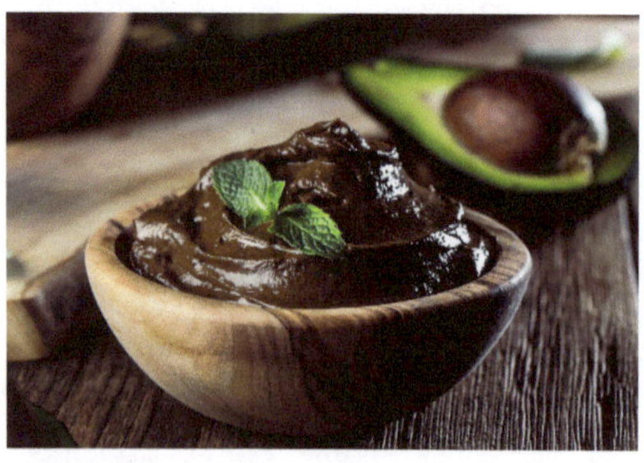

05 Banana Oatmeal Cookies

INGREDIENTS

- 2 ripe bananas, mashed
- 1 1/2 cups gluten-free rolled oats
- 1/4 cup almond butter or peanut butter
- 1/4 cup dairy-free chocolate chips or raisins (optional)
- 1 teaspoon vanilla extract
- Pinch of cinnamon (optional)

INSTRUCTIONS

1. Preheat oven to 350°F (175°C). Line a baking sheet with parchment paper.
2. In a bowl, combine mashed bananas, rolled oats, almond butter (or peanut butter), chocolate chips or raisins (if using), vanilla extract, and cinnamon (if using). Mix until well combined.
3. Drop spoonfuls of the cookie dough onto the prepared baking sheet.
4. Flatten each cookie slightly with a fork.
5. Bake for 12-15 minutes, or until cookies are golden brown.
6. Allow to cool on the baking sheet for 5 minutes, then transfer to a wire rack to cool completely.

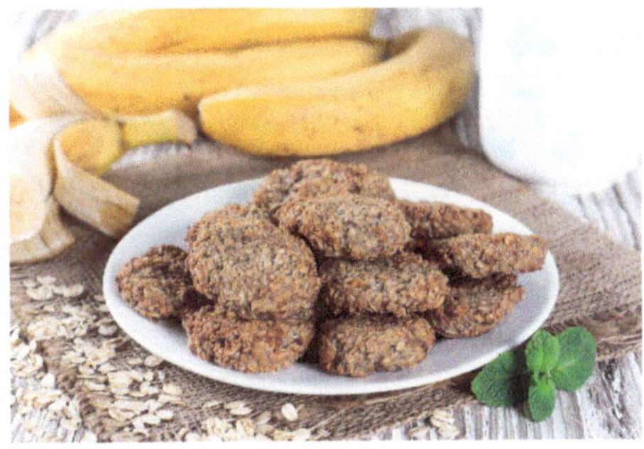

Berry Coconut Popsicles

INGREDIENTS

- 1 cup mixed berries (strawberries, blueberries, raspberries)
- 1 can (14 oz) coconut milk
- 2 tablespoons maple syrup or agave syrup (adjust to taste)
- 1/2 teaspoon vanilla extract

INSTRUCTIONS

1. In a blender, combine mixed berries, coconut milk, maple syrup (or agave syrup), and vanilla extract.
2. Blend until smooth.
3. Pour the mixture into popsicle molds.
4. Insert popsicle sticks and freeze for at least 4 hours or until completely frozen.
5. Run the molds under warm water for a few seconds to release the popsicles before serving.

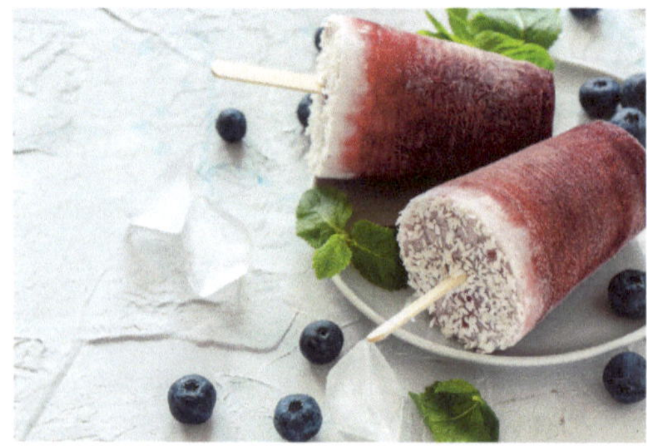

TIPS FOR SUCCESS

By incorporating these tips into your daily routine, you'll
create a sustainable and enjoyable path to better health.

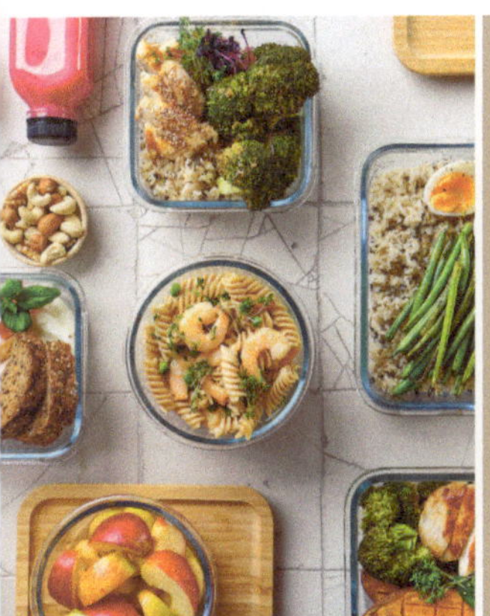

1. PLAN YOUR MEALS

Spend some time each week planning your meals and snacks. This helps you make healthier choices and reduces the temptation of convenience foods.

2. BATCH COOKING AND MEAL PREP

Dedicate a day or a few hours each week to batch cook meals and prep ingredients. This saves time during busy weekdays and ensures you have nutritious meals ready to go.

3. USE VERSATILE INGREDIENTS

Opt for ingredients that can be used in multiple dishes, such as quinoa, chickpeas, and a variety of fresh vegetables. This reduces waste and keeps your meals interesting.

4. MINDFUL EATING

Practice mindful eating by paying attention to your food choices, savoring each bite, and eating without distractions. This can help prevent overeating and promote better digestion.

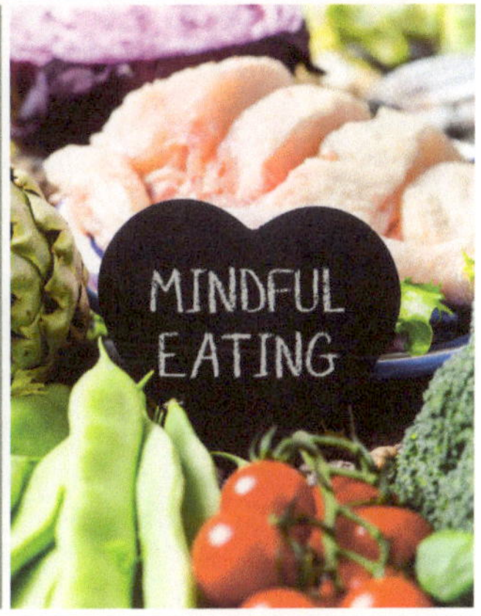

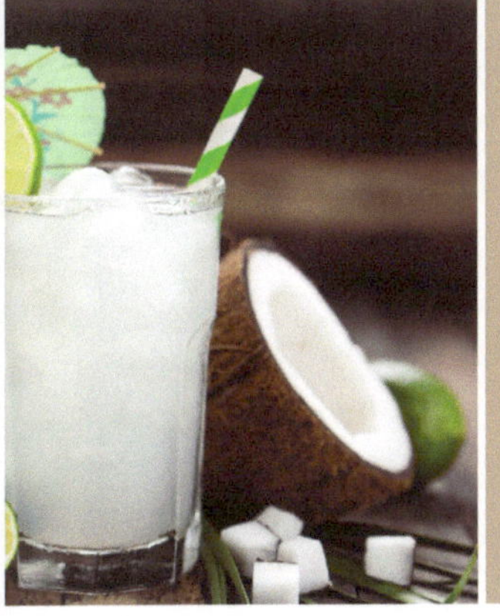

5. STAY HYDRATED

Drink plenty of water throughout the day to stay hydrated and support your body's functions. Infuse water with citrus slices, mint, or cucumber for added flavor.

6. INCORPORATE LEAN PROTEINS

Drink plenty of water throughout the day to stay hydrated and support your body's functions. Infuse water with citrus slices, mint, or cucumber for added flavor.

By implementing these insights into your routine, you're laying a strong foundation for achieving your objectives. Remember, consistent effort and persistence are the keys to reaching your desired outcomes. Stay focused, stay motivated, and embrace every step forward on your path to success!

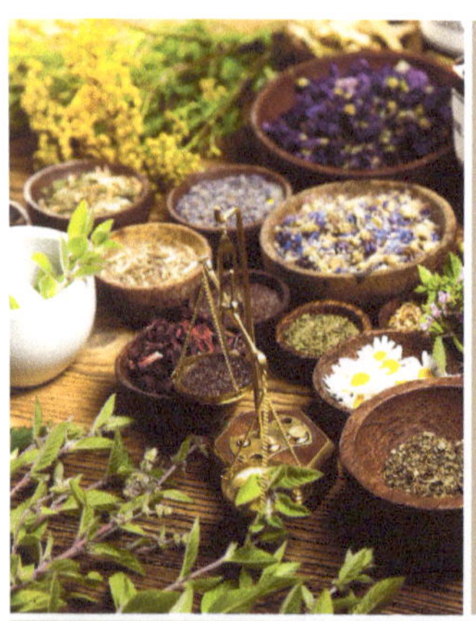

7. EXPERIMENT WITH HERBS AND SPICES

Enhance the flavor of your meals without relying on salt or unhealthy condiments by experimenting with herbs, spices, and citrus zest.

8. LISTEN TO YOUR BODY

Pay attention to hunger and fullness cues. Eat when you're hungry and stop when you're satisfied, rather than eating out of habit or boredom.

9. STAY ACTIVE

Find enjoyable ways to incorporate physical activity into your routine, whether it's a daily walk, yoga session, or workout class. Regular exercise boosts mood and supports overall health.

10. PRACTICE SELF-CARE

Take time for yourself to relax and unwind. Whether it's reading a book, taking a bath, or meditating, self-care helps reduce stress and promotes overall well-being.

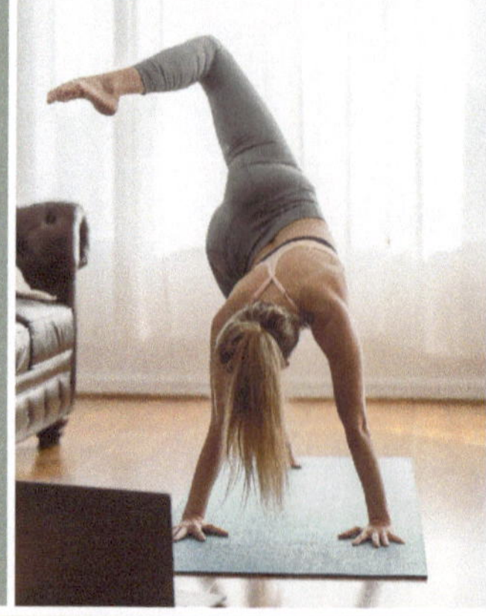

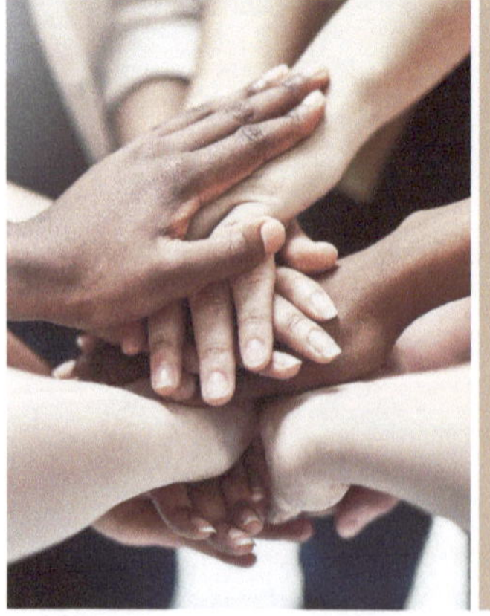

11. SEEK SUPPORT

Connect with friends, family, or online communities who share similar health goals. Having a support system can provide motivation, accountability, and encouragement on your journey.

12. CELEBRATE PROGRESS

Recognize and celebrate your achievements, no matter how small. Whether it's trying a new recipe or reaching a fitness milestone, acknowledging your progress boosts confidence and motivation.

By embracing these strategies in your daily life, you'll pave a clear and effective path toward achieving your goals. Every small step you take today contributes to significant progress over time. Stay dedicated, maintain a positive mindset, and cherish every moment of your journey!

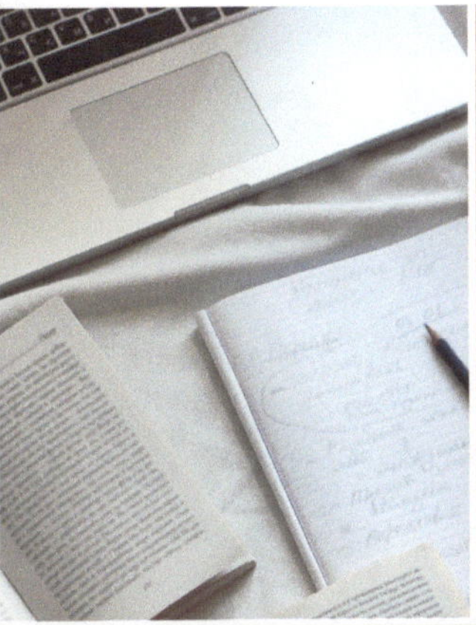

13. EDUCATE YOURSELF

Continuously learn about nutrition, healthy cooking techniques, and wellness practices. The more you know, the better equipped you'll be to make informed decisions about your health.

14. ADAPT AND ADJUST

Be flexible and willing to adapt your plan as needed. Life can be unpredictable, so having a flexible approach ensures you can maintain healthy habits in any situation.

15. ENJOY THE JOURNEY

Embrace the process of improving your health and well-being. Celebrate the positive changes you're making and find joy in nourishing your body with delicious and nutritious foods.

16. GET YOUR SLEEP/REST DAY

Recovery from workouts help to lose weight and repair the muscle you've been ripping. Make sure and improve your sleep. It is so important for your wellness journey.

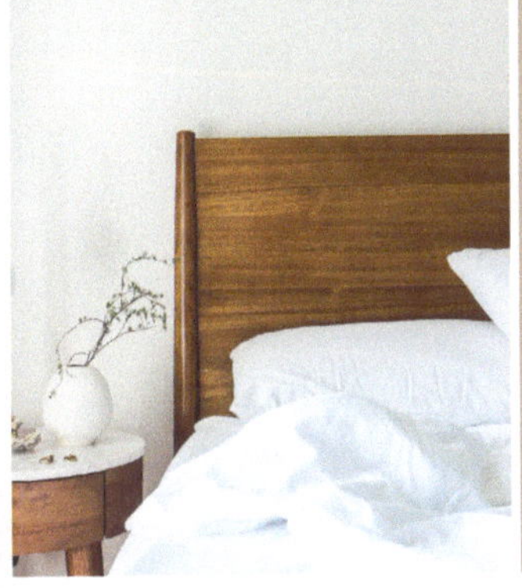

With "Wholesome Delights" as your guide, eating for weight loss and gut health has never been easier or more enjoyable. Say goodbye to restrictive diets and bland meals, and hello to a world of flavor, creativity, and vitality. Through nourishing recipes and practical tips, you've discovered how simple it can be to prioritize your well-being without sacrificing taste. Embrace the journey of transforming your health one delicious bite at a time, and savor the rewards of a balanced and vibrant lifestyle. Here's to your continued success and a future filled with wholesome delights!

Now go kick ass!!

XoXo,

Angel Rae Vigil

Non si può avere fiducia in un'umanità che perde le opere di Democrito e conserva quelle di Platone.

Erwing Schroedinger.

Prefazione

Non so neanch'io perché mi sia messo a scrivere queste pagine, in esse è la mia visione della gente e dei massimi problemi. Una cosa è certa: non sarà questo né nessun libro a cambiare lo sviluppo della società. Questa si sviluppa secondo le ragioni del ventre. Non è il politico che determina lo sviluppo della società, egli deve seguire l'onda e forse così riesce a far passare un minimo di idee controcorrente, che comunque saranno presto riassorbite. Chi è bravo a prevedere la sua evoluzione può fare carriera politica o anche farsi i soldi con gli affari. Per esempio è inutile che il finanziere si arrabbi contro l'irrazionalità delle persone quando vede una bolla speculativa: lo caricheranno di male parole, meglio che ne approfitti, sapendo che in mano ha roba che val poco e cerchi di non restare con il cerino in mano. Inoltre siccome questo libro è assai crudo non vorrei che credeste che io sia un frustrato, che sputa fiele sugli altri che sono più di lui. Pensatelo pure se vi fa piacere, io credo di essere un uomo ordinario, non disilluso perché è mai stato illuso, che osserva il mondo tenendosi in disparte. Mi piacciono gli arrivisti sociali, mi divertono i musicisti classici, i filosofi, gli umanisti, gli economisti, i bempensanti, i maestri di virtù, le persone tronfie specialmente quando si arrovellano per farsi mantenere. Non so perché siamo qui, non do molta importanza a me stesso e quindi neanche agli altri. Perché dovrei essere acido? Non ho ambizioni non appagate, perché non ho ambizioni. Vivo molto sotto le mie possibilità economiche, non perché sia ricco ma perché ho bisogno di poco. I miei interessi sono soprattutto intellettuali, non costano. Ritengo una noia ogni volta che devo comprare un'auto o un paio di pantaloni, un castigo quando devo viaggiare, non mi interessa primeggiare. Mi piace

9 798329 095050